Surviving a 5K Race

Get Running in

6 Weeks

By: John Rouda

DEDICATION

To my wife, who taught me that I can always do a little more than my mind says I can. For this, I thank you.

I love you very much.

CONTENTS

ACKNOWLEDGMENTS

Special thanks to Chris Ardis, Jacob Stancil, Michelle Jones and Chris Chandler for their fitness and running expertise over the past several years, and for the encouragement to start running in the first place. Also thanks to Team Cropduster from the Palmetto 200. I learned lots about running and having a good time from you guys.

YOUR SUPPORT & MORE INFORMATION

Thanks so much for getting this book. Please understand that ratings and reviews in Amazon are the lifeblood for a book author. Getting a good review and rating helps promote this work and more work like it. To review this book, please go to http://johnrouda.com/b/r/5k/.

To see more of my work, please visit my site at http://johnrouda.com/ and sign up for my newsletter. Thank you so much!

Also please note that 10% of all author royalties will be donated to charity.

CHAPTER 1
BEFORE YOU BEGIN

This book is not for avid runners, or those who win 5K races and just want to get better. This book is for people who either want to run their first 5K (or first in a while) or those who just want to get into 5K shape. I'm writing this for the folks that don't run, or may never have ran in the past.

I'm neither a runner nor fitness professional so please consult your physician before starting any workout program. That being said, I'm probably in no way qualified to write a fitness book. The truth of it is, I'm an IT Manager, and Computer Science Professor. So it may seem pretty strange that I'm writing about running. I know... I also thought it was strange, but the idea wouldn't go away. About 8 years ago I ran my first 5K. I was convinced that running was fun by some friends, all of whom were runners. So I decided to give it a try. After about a quarter of a mile, I decided that running sucks. I felt like my heart was beating out of my chest and my lungs couldn't find enough oxygen. I was sure that if I continued I would surely die.

Before you start following this or any 5K running guide, let me lay down some ground rules. To help you be successful.

Get fitted for running shoes.
At first you may probably feel like I did and think that you can skip this step. After all,

your expensive "running" shoes that you wear while you're not running may feel just fine and suited to the task. I skipped this step at first and started running in the same shoes that I played tennis in, played basketball in, and cut the grass wearing... that was a big mistake. After a few weeks I started getting knee pain and found that my shoes were starting to cause a mild case of runner's knee. I decided to get fitted at a local store in Charlotte, NC. They watched me run (without shoes) and took a close look at my feet using some tools that they had. Then they said I needed firm support and recommended some super expensive Saucony running shoes. I think I might have paid $129.99 for them. I now buy the same shoes online for around $60. Getting fitted is well worth the extra money for the shoes. It helps prevent injuries that typically lead to people feeling like their bodies weren't designed for running.

Start slow... slower that you feel is

necessary.

If you're like me, you probably think you can do more than you probably should. You probably put too many tasks on your plate at work, and speaking of plate, you probably put too much food on your plate at the buffet...you've got to get your money's worth. Well, with running you need to take a different mindset. As I stated earlier, I thought I was going to die after running my first quarter mile. That's because I started running way to fast. I remembered as a kid, that when you were in a race or ran, you did it fast. Well, that's just not the case anymore. You have to start slow. Start your running at around 60% of what you think your max speed is, then slow down a little. That should be the pace you start at. Over time, you can increase speed, adjust your stride, etc. However first, we want to get you moving and enjoying the run, instead of feeling like you're going to die.

Pay attention to your diet.

It's really important to know that what you put into your body, has a significant effect on what comes out of your body. Food that your body can use to convert to energy and to build muscle is important when starting any training program, especially one that burns as many calories as running. You need to eat in order to run. When I was training for my first marathon it wasn't uncommon to find me at CiCi's all you can eat pizza buffet getting more than a dozen slices of pizza after a long run. This was as I later learned was not the best thing to do, but I was starving. If I were smarter back then, I would have paid closer attention to my diet and made sure that had enough proteins and complex carbohydrates going into my body to sustain the runs. Moreover this is the part where I have to stress the importance of water. Not sports drinks...water. Drink a lot of water. Have a drink of water the night before you run, when you wake up, and of course after you've completed the run.

Take breaks and rest often.
I've found a couple of main reasons why people quit running. They either feel like their body isn't designed for running, which could be due to an injury, improper shoes, or even a bad diet. It might even be because they are burned out which generally occurs with not taking enough breaks. I don't recommend running everyday, at least not at first. Running is an acquired taste, much like drinking beer, so don't do it every day, at least not until you have acquired the taste for it to allow you to do it in moderation. When I'm training for a race, I usually will not run more than 4 times a week. And when I'm not training for a race, I usually run at least 2-3 times per week. It keeps running interesting for me and keeps me from getting burned out. I approach running now as something I "get to do" instead of something I "have to do." One note, I do have several friends that run everyday and have for years. That works great for them so

if you're one of those vaguely odd persons who go for it.

The next thing you need to do before going further in this book is to find a race. Look for one about 6 weeks out, that way you can start training today. Not tomorrow, not next week, not next month. Today. As my wife will attest, if you're like me, and probably like to put something off until tomorrow, you might as well put it off forever. I recommend going to active.com and start looking for races, or just go to Google and search for "5K race putting in your specific zip code or local area where necessary.

Surviving a 5K

CHAPTER 2
RACES

In this chapter we're going to learn about different types of races and some basic running terminology. When I was first learning to run, I would say stupid things all the time without even thinking that it sounded stupid to anyone who had any knowledge of the sport of running. For example:

Any runner: "I'm going to run the OBX Marathon"

Me: "Oh yeah, cool. How far is that?"

Any runner: "It's a full marathon"

Me: "So like 10 miles?"

Any runner: "Sigh… 26.2 miles"

Now that I participate in races frequently, I would find someone having a discussion about racing and not knowing that a marathon is 26.2 miles as ignorant, annoying and somewhat offensive to the sport. So I'll be using this chapter to educate you on some of the specifics of marathon running. First we'll start with basic running terminology.

10-K pace
10-K pace is the time per mile (pace) that a runner will run a 10 K race (6.2 miles).

5-K/8-K/10-K

The K here stands for kilometers, or 1,000 meters. A 5-K is equal to 3.1 miles; 8-K is 4.96 miles; 10-K is equal to 6.2 miles.

400 meters

The 400 meters is equivalent to a quarter mile or 1 lap around a standard track.

800 meters

The double of 400 meters as you may have already figured out is equivalent to a half-mile or 2 laps around a standard track.

Aerobic

Think of a jog. Aerobic is generally used to refer to running or any other form of exercise that offers a moderately paced cardiovascular workout to deliver the required amount of oxygen to your muscle tissues without allowing any appreciable build up of lactic acid.

Normally, you can run at a slow aerobic pace

for long periods of time, provided you have the endurance to go long distances. However, longer runs that often involve training runs are performed at an Aerobic Pace.

Anaerobic

Think of a sprint. Anaerobic is used to refer to running or other exercise that seriously gets your heart and lungs working, causing your respiratory and cardiovascular systems to deliver all or most of the oxygen required by your muscles, and fast enough that lactic acid begins to build up in your muscles, thus producing a tired, heavy feeling. Normally the pace associated with anaerobic running cannot be sustained very long.

Athena

The Athena category of runners is for weight challenged women. Typically the cutoff is set at 160lbs (which I don't think is over weight) and normally only used for big races. I'm not a fan of these types of categories, but if you see it, you'll now know what it means. The purpose of the Athena category is to give runners more opportunities to win in their class.

Chip Time

Chip time refers to a technology for detecting and recording the finishing times of all the runners in a race. It's far more accurate and can deal with the traditional problem of many runners simultaneously finishing the race as one large group. The chip time technology uses a small device that is programmed for each runner and is typically given to the runner when they check in for the race. These miniature devices can be as small as an inconspicuous bracelet or slightly larger. The chip which is generally attached to your shoe laces or worn it around your arm (depending on the type) sends a signal to another device that's typically hidden under a strip of rubber or carpet at the start and finish lines of the race. This chip automatically records your exact time at the end of the race. Usually you are asked to return the chip in to the race organizers so don't steal it.

Clydesdale
The Clydesdale category of runners is for weight challenged men. Typically the cutoff is set at 220lbs (which I don't think is over weight) and normally only used for big races. I'm not a fan of these types of categories, but if you see it, you now know what it means. The purpose is to give runners more opportunities to win in their class.

Cool-down
Slow running, jogging or even brisk walking done after a workout to loosen muscles and rid the body of lactic acid.

CR
Course record.

Cushioning
Better known as shock absorption; it's the

ability of a shoe to absorb the impact of your foot striking the ground.

DNF
Did not finish.

DNS
Did not start.

DOMS
Delayed Onset Muscle Soreness. A type of muscle soreness that normally peaks about 48 hours after an intense workout or run.

Elite Runner
A runner who is super fast and has reached the highest level in his sport.

Fartlek
Sometimes called intervals. A fartlek is a variable pace running technique which includes a mixture of slow running, running at a moderate speed, and short, fast sprints. Fartlek training is a way to increase speed

and endurance and I've found it's great for runners just starting to add distance.

"Hitting the Wall"
During a race when your muscles become depleted and a feeling of fatigue hits you; that's when you "hit the wall." It's an awful feeling where you feel like you can't run anymore. I "hit the wall" during the 2007 OBX Marathon on mile 22. It's rough.

Intervals
A training exercise in which short and fast repetitions (sprints) are alternated with slow intervals of jogging for recovery; interval training can help build both speed and endurance. I would recommend intervals after building a 5K base when trying to increase your distance or your speed.

Junk Miles
In my opinion and for this book, there is no such thing. Some more experienced runners will say that junk miles are runs at an easy

pace put into a training program so that you can reach a weekly or monthly mileage total. They often serve as recovery from harder, more intense workouts. I believe that all miles count and help you, especially when you're just starting running or working to complete your first 5 or 10K.

Lactic Acid
A substance which forms in your muscles as a result of the breakdown of glucose. Lactic acid is associated with muscle soreness and muscle fatigue.

LSD
A popular hallucinogen from the 70s... just kidding. LSD stands for "Long, Slow Distance," which refers to longer, easier (slower paced) training runs. These runs can help when training for races, both long and short. For example, an LSD for a 7 minute per mile 5K racer might be a 9 minute 5 miler LSD.

Marathon
A 26.2 mile race. This race got its name in 490 B.C., when a Greek soldier name Philippides ran the distance from the battle of Marathon to Athens, where he died after the Greek victory over the Persians. The distance was supposedly 26.2 miles.

Master
Also called a Veteran. A Master is a runner over the age of 40.

Maximum Heart Rate
The maximum heart-rate achieved during a specified workout.

"Metric Mile"
This used to confuse the crap out of me. But basically it's just 1500 meters; the international distance closest to the imperial mile used in racing.

Mile
I hope you know what a mile is, but if you

don't its 1609 meters, 5280 feet, or 1760 yards.

Negative Splits
Running the second half of a race faster than the first half, or more specifically, running later miles faster than earlier miles. For example, during a 5K, if you might run 10 minute for your 1st mile, 9:30 for your second, and 9 for your third.

NR
National record.

Overpronation
Usually associated with flat feet, but it's where you excessively roll the foot while walking or running. Overpronation is an often associated with many running injuries.

Pick-Ups
Quick burst of speed done during a run. These are normally done in shorter durations than fartleks. Pick-ups are just

away to add some excitement to what could become a boring run.

Plyometrics
Any jumping exercise. Usually highly intense and a great form of cardiovascular workout.

Pronation
Pronation is a normal and necessary motion for walking or running. It is the inward roll of the foot as the arch of the foot collapses.

PR/PB
Personal record/personal best.

Ride
The ability of a shoe to give you a smooth transfer of a runner's weight from heel-strike to toe-off... like a car, giving you a smooth ride. A shoe's ride is a very subjective quality, but runners know it when a shoe has a good ride.

Runner's High

A feeling of bliss, joy, and well-being associated with intense running. This is apparently due to a rush of endorphins. For more on this, I highly recommend watching Robin Williams' stand-up on Runners high. See more at
 http://runbikehike.us/runnershigh/ .

Running Economy
This is how much oxygen your body uses when you run. When you improve your running economy, you are able to run while using a smaller amount of oxygen.

Splits
Splits refers to your times or pace at mile markers or other pre-planned checkpoints along the way.

Stability
The ability of a shoe to resist excessive foot motion and hold up to stress during the run.

Strides

Strides are short, fast, and controlled runs of 50 to 150 meters. Strides can be used for both training and to warm up before a race. During training they are used to build speed and efficiency.

Taper
Runners usually cut back mileage (or taper down their distance) one week to three weeks (depending on race distance) before a big race. Tapering helps muscles rest so that they are ready for peak performance on race day.

Target Heart Rate
The range your heart rate reaches during aerobic training, that enables you to get the most out of your workout. Your target heart rate will vary.

Tempo Runs
A type of training run where you usually run 20 to 30 minutes in length, at 10 to 15 seconds per mile slower than your 10-K race

pace.

Toebox
The front part of a shoe. A wide toebox allows plenty of room for the toes to spread.

Veteran
A term similar to a master in the U.S. According to the IAAF, men become "veterans" on their 40th birthday and women become "veterans" on their 35th birthday.

Warm-up
Five to fifteen minutes of easy jogging/walking before a race or a workout. The purpose of a warm-up is to raise your heart rate so your muscles are looser and to prevent injury.

WR
World record.

Surviving a 5K

CHAPTER 3
WEEK 1

Week one is going to be your hardest week, especially if you've never run before, or if you're just starting out running. During this week you'll need to be focusing on two things, finishing your run, and running consistently. During week one we want you to start building a habit of running. Make your body regret the days you don't run. There are a couple of things at work inside your body as you start running. First your muscles begin to strengthen.

In order for your muscles to grow, you must tear them down. Working out tears muscle cells down, allowing them to repair themselves making you stronger. Just as a farmer must prune a plant in order for it to produce its best fruit, your body does the same thing.

So I took 6 months off from running before writing this book.   That was actually harder to do than you might think.   Running consistently becomes a habit after you do it for several weeks, and just like the coffee habit, you get addicted. And when you quit running for a while, you feel bad about yourself and you feel the urge to run to feel better. At least that's how I feel. My body misses that runners high. I took the time off for 2 reasons, first I had a new baby son that stole my sleep (love that boy), and second I wanted to be able to write about how it feels when you're starting over or starting new, so that you'll know you're not alone.

The first mile walking is important. It loosens your muscles and makes you feel good about yourself, then the running starts. The first run is your hardest. About a minute in, I feel my lungs burning, my heart is pounding and my brain is telling me that there is no way in heck I can do this; I'm definitely not qualified to be writing about running. You'll be thinking similar thoughts... that's okay, it's normal. You can do this. Just keep counting down the time. One thing that helps me is finding something else to focus on. I often find that listen to audio books or podcasts quite helpful. You might listen to music. Do what works for you.

Don't let Saturday fool you. It sounds easy doing the 10 run/walk intervals, but 1 minute recovery time for a 30 second run isn't much time. I tried sprinting this out for the first few, then it ended as a jog. I probably would have done better if I started slower on those runs during the run/walk section.

Steven Covey so famously states in his Seven Habits of Highly Effective People to "Start with the end in mind." Six weeks from now you will be running a 5K race. Never lose focus of the goal, and keep the end in mind.

Beginner's Schedule – Week 1:

Monday: Walk briskly for 1 mile. Run 2 minutes every half mile until you reach 3.5 total miles. Walk 0.5 mile.

Tuesday: Walk 3-5 miles.

Wednesday: Off – enjoy it!

Thursday: Walk 1 mile. Run 3 minutes every half mile until you reach 3.5 miles. Walk 0.5 mile.

Friday: Off – Don't party too hard. You've got a tough run tomorrow.

Saturday: Walk 3-5 miles, including 10 run/walk intervals (run 30 seconds, walk 1 minutes) in the last mile.

Sunday: Off – get your church on.

Week Total: 16-20 miles – That's crazy! You went more than 15 miles in your 1st week! Congrats!

For the experienced runner...

Every week I'll have a schedule for those that find that the beginner's schedule isn't stretching their will power enough.

So what makes you an experienced runner? Well I would consider an experienced runner someone who has ran a 5k in the last year. Someone would could run/walk 3 miles and only be slightly sore in the morning. Again, this book is NOT for everyday runners, so if you're an everyday runner by all means, read and enjoy, however you might want to consider donating this book to a friend that doesn't run, but should.

Experienced Schedule - Week 1:

Monday: Run 5 minutes, walk 1 min – repeat 3 times
Tuesday: Rest or cross-train
Wednesday: Run 6 minutes, walk 1 min – repeat 3 times
Thursday: Rest
Friday: Run 7 minutes, walk 1 min – repeat 3 times
Saturday: Rest or cross-train
Sunday: Rest

CHAPTER 4
WEEK 2

Our goal for week 2 is to keep doing what we started in week 1 and make running become more of a habit. As you know, habits can be hard to break. There are good habits, like brushing your teeth in the morning, and bad habits, like smoking. We want running consistently to become one of our good habits.

Making a habit.
There are 3 steps to creating any good habit

and 3 "R's" in the framework for habit change. If you're interested in more about habits, please checkout "The Power of Habit" by Charles Duhigg.

3 R's of Habit Change
1. **Reminder** (Create a trigger that starts the new behavior). For me, this is the hardest part. I'm so inconsistent when it comes to routine, that I found it hard to have a solid time that I will always run. For most people its all about timing. Either they run after work, or in the morning before work, or at lunch. However, for me, I found that I run when I want to… not consistently in the morning, or in the evening. This is not good. Creating a reminder for me, was tough. When I was training for the OBX Marathon, getting into the habit of running was really tough, and its all because I didn't have a good reminder. After several weeks, I finally got into a

pattern of running. Looking back on it, it all happened when I made up my mind to run right after work. This "reminder" triggered my routine and helped me make running a habit.

2. **Routine** (The behavior or action your creating/changing). This is the easy part. Start running. Your routine is just following the schedule outlined in this book. I am including a simple chart at the end of the book that you can follow along with a link you can print to just see the schedule.

3. **Reward** (the benefit for the behavior). This is the fun part. Give yourself a reward. For me candy, food, etc usually works. Most of the time it was ice cream. I'm sure that most health professionals will cringe at reading this, but it's the truth, at least for me. However, sometimes I didn't reward myself with treats, yet, as I

have found that running itself has become a sort of reward. I feel good when I run, good about myself both physically and mentally. I know that the same feeling will happen to you.

These 3 R's create what Duhigg calls a "habit loop."

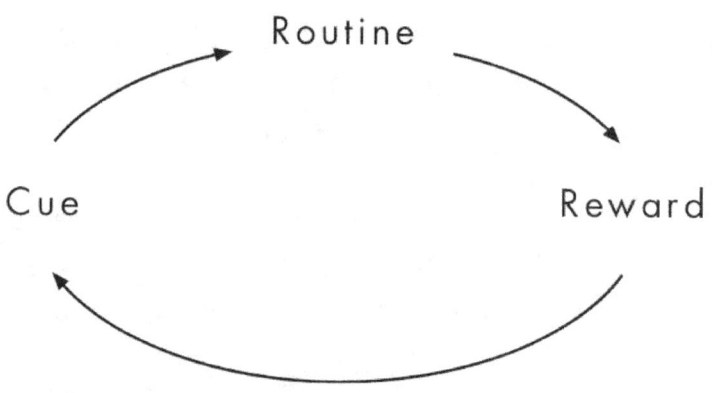

3 Steps for creating a new habit

1. **Set your reminder** – This can be a timing thing, like running in the

morning, lunch, or after work.

2. **Follow the plan in the book** – This step is pretty easy. ☺

3. **Choose your reward** – Hopefully the act of running will become your reward, but if you need a little motivation to get started, I recommend sugar free or reduced fat ice cream.

Beginner's Schedule – Week 2:

Monday: Walk 1.5 miles. Run 5 minutes, walk 5 minutes; do 3 times. Walk 1-2 miles.
Tuesday: Walk 3-5 miles.
Wednesday: Off
Thursday: Repeat Week 1 Thursday.
Friday: Off
Saturday: Repeat Week 2 Monday.
Sunday: Off
Week Total: 18-20 miles

Experienced Schedule - Week 2:

Monday: Run 7 minutes, walk 1 min – repeat 3 times
Tuesday: Rest or cross-train
Wednesday: Run 8 minutes, walk 1 min – repeat 3 times
Thursday: Rest
Friday: Run 9 minutes mile, walk 1 min – repeat 3 times
Saturday: Rest or cross-train
Sunday: Off

Chapter 5
Week 3

Finding your motivation. I've given countless classes and talks on motivation. How to motivate yourself at work, your team, and your students. Motivating yourself to run however is a different story. There are no financial or career aspects to look forward to. This I found much harder, but I have been able to find some connections between the two and I hope my advice below helps you keep your motivation for running.

If you're like me, by week 3 running is starting to get boring. You're probably running the same course repeatedly, seeing the same trees, houses, etc. This is the time that I would recommend changing your environment. I once experimented with this at work. I changed my team's environment by removing all cube walls to see if it would spark some motivation. I got the idea after hearing the story of Doug Dietz.

Doug Dietz is a brilliant engineer. He makes medical devices, specifically MRI machines. His machines have saved thousands of lives over the years and he is very proud of his work. One day, he decided to leave his office and go and see some of his machines in action. This change of environment inspired him to make a huge, yet simple, break through in the design of MRI machines for children. You see, when Doug was visiting the hospitals he noticed that nearly 80% of all the pediatric patients had to be sedated to use the MRI machine. They saw it as a scary place and didn't want anything to do with it. This was disturbing for Doug. In his efforts to create a more pleasant experience for the patient he added some paint and a new designs for the exterior and created what you see below. He turned the machine on the left, from a chilling place, into a place of wonder and excitement. Now, less than 20% of pediatric patients that use Doug's new machines need to be sedated.

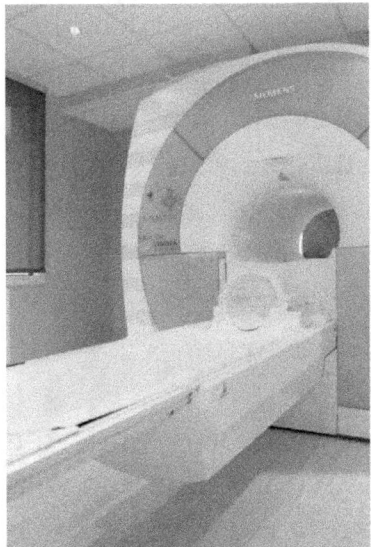
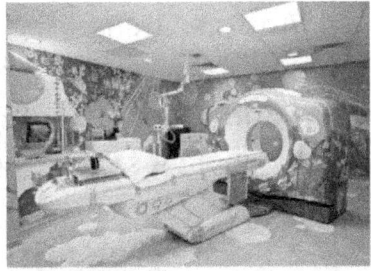
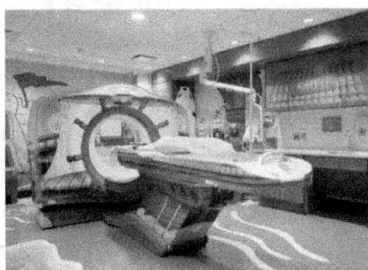

Doug was inspired and motivated to make these changes by changing his environment. I think changing your running environment can do the same thing for you. I recommend staying off the treadmill (unless a truly last option) and trying something new each week. Maybe run the same course in reverse, or try a different neighborhood near by. Go to the local college or university and run there. The options are truly endless.

Another thing I found that keeps me excited for a run is what I do when I run. I listen to audio books. Okay, okay, I'm a nerd, but it really helps me stay stoked about running. I try to find a few really good audio books, and discipline myself to only listen to them when I run. This way, if I want to find out what happens next, I have to run.

My last piece of advice for getting motivated to run, is to find someone to either run with you or hold you accountable. The former is always better, because its great to have company while running. But its easy to disappoint your self, but much harder to let someone else down. If someone is running with you, or holding you accountable for running, you feel obligated to them to keep running. I recommend finding one or more people that will run with you, and give them a copy of this book as a gift for agreeing to help you through the journey.

Beginner's Schedule – Week 3:
Monday: Walk 1.5 miles. Run 10 minutes, walk 5-7 minutes, run 10 minutes, walk 5-7 minutes.
Tuesday: Walk 3-5 miles.
Wednesday: Off
Thursday: Walk 3-5 miles.
Friday: Off
Saturday: Walk 1.5 miles. Run 10 minutes, walk 5 minutes, run 5 minutes, walk 5 minutes, run 10 minutes, walk 5-10 minutes.
Sunday: Off
Week Total: 16-20 miles

Experienced Schedule - Week 3:
Monday: Run 10 minutes, walk 1 min – repeat 2 times
Tuesday: Cross-train
Wednesday: Run 12 minutes, walk 1 min – repeat 2 times
Thursday: Rest
Friday: Run 13 minutes, walk 1 min – repeat 2 times
Saturday: Rest or cross-train

Sunday: Rest

Surviving a 5K

CHAPTER 6

WEEK 4

Making it stick

You're more than half way through your 5K training. Way to go! I hope by now that you're beginning to feel more comfortable running. You should be able to complete the training and not feel like you're going to die, but if you do, its okay. Your breathing should be a bit better, and your legs probably don't feel like Jell-O when you finish a training run either.   These are all signs that you're getting better.   You're actually doing this. You are now a runner.

One of my favorite quotes from Robin Sharma, author of Extraordinary Leadership and The Monk Who Sold His Ferrari is that, "small daily improvements over time lead to stunning results." You may not see it now, but if you look back on where you started, your results should be stunning.   You've been making small improvements on every training run.   Sometimes you might not see it, because small contributions are easily overlooked, but the sum of those contributions makes a big impact.

During your runs this week I want you to think about the race.   Think about the goal of completing the 5K.   By now you've made a habit of running.   The first mile may still be hard for you... its still the hardest for me, but its probably not has hard as it was week 1. Try to focus on running efficiently.   One of the biggest reasons that runners aren't efficient while running is because their muscles are weak. If your muscles are weak, then you compensate your form to make up for the weakness. We do the same thing in life. If you're not good at talking in person, you probably email more. If you're a terrible typist, you probably make more phone calls, etc. Running is no different. There are many different things you can do to improve your strength. Below are a few exercises that I recommend to improve strength, which will lead to more efficient running.

Push-ups

One of the best bodyweight exercises in my opinion is the push-up. While most people wouldn't make that connection between push-ups and running, it is a match made in heaven. Push-ups not only strengthen your arms (which will get sore over long runs if not in shape) but they strengthen your core which helps you have good posture while running and a necessity if you want to be efficient.

Steps to do a push-up
•   Get in a starting push-up position with hands flat on the ground and legs together (spread legs apart to make it easier)
•   Lower your body down to 1-inch from the ground
•   Explode up so hard that your hands leave the ground
• For advanced folks, try clapping.

Squats

While push-ups are the best bodyweight exercise, squats are the most fundamenta exercise for strengthening your legs. By doing squats, you will build strength and endurance in your all major lower-body muscles (glutes, hamstrings, quads and calves).

Steps to do a squat

• While standing, bend your hips and knees until your legs are at a 90 degree angle; keep your back arched throughout the movement.

• While in the lower squat position, explode upward to the starting position and repeat.

Mountain Climbers

No, you won't be climbing up a mountain but it will feel like you have when you do this exercise right. This is a great tool to use to burn fat, build muscle and boost endurance levels. It may not be as tough as climbing a mountain, but it will help prepare your for your race.

Steps to do mountain climbers

- With your hands shoulder width apart on the floor (in a push-up position)
- Keeping the push-up position, put one leg forward underneath your torso while keeping other leg straight back
- Alternate legs back and forth as if you are running in place

Beginner's Schedule – Week 4:

Monday: Walk 1 mile. Run 3 minutes, walk 2 minutes; do a total of 10 times. Walk 5 minutes.

Tuesday: Walk 1 mile. Run 15 minutes, walk 5 minutes, run 15 minutes, walk 5 minutes.

Wednesday: Off

Thursday: Walk 1 mile. Run 5 minutes, walk 2 minutes; do that 7-minute sequence 5 times. Walk 5 minutes.

Friday: Off

Saturday: Walk 1 mile. Run 10 minutes, walk 5 minutes; do that 15-minute sequence 3 times.

Sunday: Off

Week Total: 17.5 miles

Experienced Schedule - Week 4:

Monday: Run 15 minutes, walk 1 min - repeat 2 times

Tuesday: Cross-train

Wednesday: Run 17 minutes, walk 1 min, run 7 min

Thursday: Rest

Friday: Run 19 minutes, walk 1 min, run 7 min

Saturday: Rest or cross-train

Sunday: Rest

CHAPTER 7
WEEK 5

You're almost there. Finish strong. Now that you've been running for 4 weeks, what's another week? Just finish strong. After a month of solid running its easy to want to take a break and take a few days off. Don't do it. What I've found is that when you take a couple of days off... a couple of days turns can quickly turn into a couple of weeks. Just don't do it. I hope by now, you're feeling good about what you've done and you should have a solid routine for running. It should be a habit now.

I expect that you're far healthier than you were when you started 4 weeks ago and I bet if you tried the week 1 training again it would seem like a piece of cake. Okay, time to get into the guts of week 5.

Running should feel good to you now. You should be enjoying yourself while you're out there, however, if you're like me, you may be getting bored. I recommend listening to an audio book or a Ted Talk while doing your runs. It helps the time go by. To see some of what I listen to while I run, check out http://runbikehike.us/entertainment/ .

I expect that you've already started seeing some changes in your body by now. You may not experience any significant weight loss as you're likely to have a much larger appetite. This means your body is burning more fuel and wants more to replace it. This might be a good time to skip ahead to chapter 9 and read about nutrition. I'm not an expert and I seldom consider myself as the person with a health diet. I do however recommend using a tool like "My Fitness Pal" to keep track of what you eat. It's pretty cool and has some of the best tools to let you know when you're eating too much fat or sodium. Furthermore you can use the app on your phone and scan barcodes of foods that you're eating. It also keeps track of your water intake as well as tracks your fitness. Over all it's a great tool.

This week at church my pastor, Pastor Steven Furtick, was talking about "The Power of Same." He said, *If you resist the monotonous, you'll miss the miraculous."* I think the same applies to running. If you don't stick with it and keep being consistent in your efforts, you'll never get the glory of finishing the race with the time you're aiming for. Another awesome quote from the sermon that fully relates to this book and your training is "It's the process you'll resist that creates the results that you want." If you want to hear more from this and other sermons by Pastor Steven Furtick at Elevation Church visit http://elevationchurch.org/sermons/ .

Beginner's Schedule – Week 5:

Monday: Walk 1 mile. Run 3 minutes, walk 2 minutes; do that 5-minute sequence a total of 10 times. Walk 5 minutes.

Tuesday: Walk 1 mile. Run 20 minutes, walk 5 minutes, run 20 minutes, walk 5 minutes.

Wednesday: Off

Thursday: Walk 1 mile. Run 5 minutes, walk 2 minutes; do that 7-minute sequence 5 times. Walk 5 minutes.

Friday: Off

Saturday: Walk 1 mile. Run 15 minutes, walk 5 minutes; do that 20-minute sequence 3 times.

Sunday: Off

Week Total: 20 miles

Experienced Schedule - Week 5:

Monday: Run 20 minutes, walk 1 min, run 6 min

Tuesday: Cross-train

Wednesday: Run 24 minutes

Thursday: Rest

Friday: Run 26 minutes

Saturday: Rest or cross-train
Sunday: Rest

CHAPTER 8
WEEK 6

Race week baby!

You've made... well, almost. It's your race week. This is the week you've been waiting for. So we'll work hard early on, then take it slow and finish strong with the race on Saturday. Take it easy this week. Don't try to run too hard or too fast. You're close to the finish line, you don't want to screw it up while trying to be a hot-shot and running too hard. Keep it nice and slow this week. You can run hard on Saturday.

This week nutrition is really important. So please, skip ahead to chapter 9. You've probably heard many people talk about "carb loading" before a race. This is a 5K, carb loading isn't necessary. Carb loading is more important during endurance races like triathlons and marathons, however, I still use it as an excuse to eat a big pasta meal in the middle of the week. ⍰ You really don't want to carb load right before the race. If your race is on Saturday, I would recommend eating heavy on Wednesday or Thursday but no later. You don't want a belly ache while you're running.

The night before the race, drink lots of water. The last thing you want is to be dehydrated during a race. I've noticed upwards of a minute difference on my per mile splits when I'm hydrated versus dehydrated. So keep the water flowing and avoid alcohol and coffee the night before, which is tough for me because I usually drink a cup of coffee every evening (I know, I'm weird). You also want to get a really good night's sleep before your race. You always perform better when you get some sleep.

For most races you can either pick up your race packet the day before or the morning of the race. If you got it the day before, make sure you have everything you need for the race and don't forget your bib (your race number) or any timing chips that they give you. If you don't have your timing chip, then you're not going to get an official time.

The morning of the race be sure you get up early and have a good breakfast. I don't recommend chocolate chip pancakes here. Maybe get some fruit and protein with lots of water. Give yourself time to digest your food before the race. Don't eat a big breakfast at 7:30am when the race starts at 8:00am. That will just lead to cramps and bad run. Be sure you dress for the weather too, if its raining, you'll likely want a change of clothes and shoes for when you finish up the race.

While you're running the 5K, don't try push yourself too hard. I'd estimate that half of the people that run their first 5K go out too fast during the first mile and have little or nothing left for the last 2 miles. You should try to keep the pace you've been training at for at least the first 2 miles and see how you feel. If you feel good at that pace after 2 miles, try to bump it up a little for the last one. One thing I usually do is try to make my last 1.1 mile faster than my first 1 mile. Most GPS apps like Run Keeper, Map My Run, and Run Bike Hike allow you to keep track of your split paces. That way you know how fast you run each mile.

Be sure not to let up as you approach and cross the finish line. Finish strong. Then once you're done, enjoy yourself. Most races have snacks and drinks at the end. They also do an awards ceremony. I recommend staying for it if you can. It's usually a good time, even if you're not winning anything.

Beginner's Schedule – Week 6:

Monday: Walk 1 mile. Run 3 minutes, walk 2 minutes; do that 5-minute sequence a total of 10 times. Walk 5 minutes.

Tuesday: Walk 1 mile. Run 25 minutes, walk 5 minutes, run 25 minutes, walk 5 minutes.

Wednesday: Off

Thursday: Walk 1 mile. Run 5 minutes, walk 2 minutes; do that 7-minute sequence 5 times. Walk 5 minutes.

Friday: Off

Saturday: Race Day!

Sunday: Celebrate

Week Total: 22.5 miles

Experienced Schedule - Week 6:

Monday: Run 28 minutes

Tuesday: Rest or cross-train

Wednesday: Run 30 minutes

Thursday: Rest

Friday: Run 20 minutes

Saturday: Rest

Sunday: Race! Run 3.1 miles

CHAPTER 9
NUTRITION

Getting through several weeks of grueling, high-intense training is 50% what it takes to be 5K race ready. The other 50% is consuming proper foods and beverages along with following the other helpful tips below.

Drink at least half of your bodyweight in water ounces

It is nearly impossible to fully function without drinking water. Since our body is made up of about 70% water, it makes sense that we drink an adequate amount of it per day. While it has numerous benefits, the main benefit of drinking water is it helps cleanse your system; thus, making it easier for your body to do things such as burn fat. So if you know that weight loss would help your preparation efforts for the mud race, then start drinking more water. At least aim to drink half of your bodyweight in ounces. For instance, if you weigh 180lbs, then aim for about 90 ounces of water per day. Note: Please drink water before, during and after your 5K race and all training activities; especially if you're competing in a hot climate. Getting dehydrated on race day is not what you want!

Eat an adequate amount of slow-digesting

carbs per day

While carbs may get a bad rep in most of today's fad diet books, you need slow-digesting carbs to have energy to run through your training days. Here is the list of slow-digesting carbs:

- Fresh fruit (apples, oranges, grapes, etc.)

- Non-starchy vegetables (spinach, kale, tomatoes, broccoli, cauliflower, cucumber onions, asparagus, carrots, mushrooms, etc.)

- Sweet potatoes

- Nuts (walnuts, macadamia nuts, pecans, etc.)

- Natural nut butter

- Steel-cut oats

Slow-digesting carbs are perfect to eat before every 5K race training session and the day of the race. Unlike fast-digesting carbs (candy, cookies, sugars, etc.), they provide a steady dose of carbs throughout the day in which helps maintain high energy levels, i.e. no crash.

Aim for at least 3 to 4 servings of milk per week

Got milk? I'm sure you know that milk supports strong, healthy bones, which will improve injury prevention while running. Not only that, but milk aids in weight loss as well. In a research study, people who ate a reduced-calorie diet that was rich in dairy (including milk) versus those who ate a diet low in dairy, the people who consumed high quantities of dairy lost the most weight. So if you need to lose weight before race day, then milk will do your body good! Milk is also a great source of protein which will help build those leg muscles.

Don't compare yourself to other runners

The last thing you want to do is try to compare yourself to others who have been running 5k races for years. As a newbie, you simply need to focus on doing YOUR best. You can't expect to be the best racer at your first race. Michael Jordan wasn't considered the greatest basketball player as a rookie. He had to earn that title by putting in consistent, high-quality effort throughout his career. So if you expect to be the best (or one of the best) 5K racer, be prepared to continually put your best effort into your training. Or, if your like me, just enjoy watching the elites run and be happy that you are physically able to complete the race. Remember, our goal is finishing strong, not winning.

Enjoy yourself

Through all the time and miles that you put into preparing for and participating in this 5K race, remember to enjoy yourself. Too many individuals forget that these races were created to have fun. So relax and have some fun.

ABOUT THE AUTHOR

John Rouda is an IT professional and Computer Science Professor. Currently, he manages a team of web developers and teaches as an adjunct faculty member at York Technical College and at Winthrop University. John currently has over 50 mobile apps in the Apple Appstore as well as over 20 in the Google Play Marketplace. He holds two master degrees, one in Business Administration and one in Computer Science. His first book is "What's HTML?" a guide to learning HTML in only 4 hours. Visit http://whatshtml.com/book/

John is married to a wonderful wife and has a beautiful family that he dearly loves. You can find out more about John at http://www.johnrouda.com/ or follow him on twitter @johnrouda.

Surviving a 5K

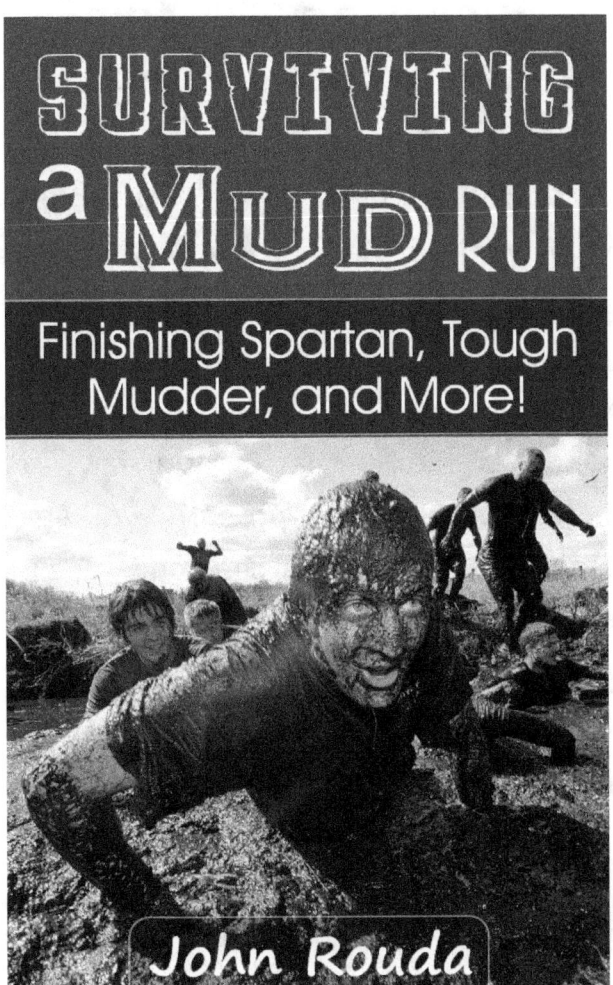

Surviving a Mud Run!
Bonus book excerpt...

So you got 8 weeks till you run your first Tough Mudder, Spartan Race or whatever mud race you signed up for. So are you physically and mentally ready to that? Will you easily make it to the finish line or make a mud face (i.e. fall flat on your face in the mud)? Depending how prepared you are will dictate your success in the mud race. This week 1 and 2 training guide will make sure you start off on the right foot. So if you ready to "murder" a Tough Mudder race or "spank" a Spartan Race, then proceed!

Training Frequency

You will train 4 days per week. In this sample training guideline, the training days at the gym will be on Monday, Tuesday, Thursday, and Friday. Wednesday, Saturday and Sunday are active rest days. Chose whatever 4 days you have at least 45 minutes to 1 hour to train.

Exercise Guidelines

Some exercises that are performed with weights will based off a percentage of your 1-rep max (1RM). For example, you are prescribed to do bench press for 3 x 10 (75% 1RM) with 90 seconds rest. That means that you do 10 reps for 3 sets with a weight that is 75% of your 1 rep max and rest 90 seconds between sets. Each exercise will help engage movements that you will likely have to perform in a mud race.

Week 1 Training Routine (Monday)
Warm-up Routine (do each exercise in order for 1 minute)

- Jog in place

- Jumping Jacks

- Lunge Walks

- Arm Circles

Exercise :	Dumb-bell Chest Press	Barbell Squats	Pushups	Burpees	Jump Rope
Sets / Reps:	3 x 10 reps	3 x 10 reps	3 x 20 reps	3 x 15 reps	5 x 30 secs
Rest time:	90 secs	90 secs	60 secs	60 secs	30 secs
% of 1RM:	70%	70%	Body weight	Body weight	Body weight

To read more and learn more about its release date, go to http://johnrouda.com/mudrun/

YOUR SUPPORT & MORE INFORMATION

Thanks so much for getting this book. Please understand that ratings and reviews in Amazon are the lifeblood for a book author. Getting a good review and rating helps promote this work and more work like it. To review this book, please go to http://johnrouda.com/b/r/5k/.

To see more of my work, please visit my site at http://johnrouda.com/ and sign up for my newsletter. Thank you so much!

Also please note that 10% of all author royalties will be donated to charity.

www.ingramcontent.com/pod-product-compliance
Lightning Source LLC
Chambersburg PA
CBHW071222280526
45787CB00002B/760